HOW TO MAKE NATURAL SOAP FOR BEGINNERS

ESSENTIAL GUIDE ON HOW TO MAKE SOAP FROM SCRATCH, NATURAL SOAP MAKING FOR BEGINNERS

Yonani Frunce

TABLE OF CONTENT

INTRODUCTION

Welcome to the arena of herbal herbal soap making! Whether you are seeking to create a more fit alternative to commercial soaps, explore a brand new hobby, or even start a small enterprise, this e book will manual you thru every step of the manner. By the quit, you may not most effective apprehend how to make your very own soap however additionally admire the blessings of the use of herbal components.

THE BENEFITS OF HOMEMADE HERBAL SOAP

In latest years, there was a growing recognition of the chemical compounds and synthetic ingredients found in many commercial skincare merchandise. Homemade herbal soap offers a herbal, green alternative that is gentle for your pores and skin and loose from dangerous components. Using natural ingredients lets in you to tailor every batch in your nonpublic desires and choices, developing a product this is as specific as you are.

WHAT YOU'LL LEARN

This ebook is designed with novices in mind, presenting a comprehensive introduction to cleaning soap making.

1. Understanding Soap and Its Ingredients: Learn about the fundamental components of soap, consisting of oils, lye, and herbal additives, and how they work together to create a cleansing bar.

2. Essential Tools and Equipment: Discover the equipment and safety gadget you will want to set up your soap making workspace.

3. The Basics of Soap Making: Explore different soap making methods consisting of bloodless process, warm procedure, and soften and pour, with step through step commands for each.

Four. Incorporating Herbs into Your Soap: Find out the way to put together and use herbs on your cleaning soap, from making herbal infusions to including crucial oils.

5. Creating Your Own Recipes: Gain the information to formulate your very own soap recipes, balancing cleansing, moisturizing, and lathering homes.

6. Coloring and Scenting Your Soap: Learn a way to use natural colorants and important oils to create superbly coloured and fragrances soaps.

7. Advanced Techniques and Tips: Master extra complex cleaning soap making techniques inclusive of swirling, layering, and embedding, and discover ways to troubleshoot commonplace troubles.

Eight. Curing, Storing, and Packaging: Understand the significance of curing cleaning soap, how to store it properly, and innovative packaging thoughts.

9. Going Beyond the Basics: Explore uniqueness soaps, seasonal subject matters, or even how to show your interest into a enterprise.

10. Resources and References: Access a list of encouraged books, web sites, suppliers, and soap making groups for similarly gaining knowledge of and help.

INTRODUCTION TO THE BENEFITS OF NATURAL, SELF MADE CLEANING SOAP.

Welcome to the captivating international of natural, self made soap making! This adventure isn't always simplest about crafting a lovely and practical product however additionally approximately embracing a lifestyle that values fitness, sustainability, and creativity. Let's explore the several advantages of creating your personal herbal herbal cleaning soap and why it's a splendid choice for you and your family.

HEALTH BENEFITS

One of the most compelling motives to switch to self made cleaning soap is the fitness advantages it gives. Commercial soaps often incorporate artificial chemical substances, preservatives, and artificial fragrances that can aggravate the skin and cause allergies. In contrast, home made soaps are crafted with natural elements which are gentle on the pores and skin. By using plant based totally oils, butters, and natural components, you could create soaps that nourish and moisturize, helping to keep wholesome and hydrated pores and skin.

No Harmful Chemicals: Homemade soap is unfastened from harsh chemicals like sodium lauryl sulfate (SLS), parabens, and that are not unusual in commercial merchandise

Tailored to Your Skin Needs: You can customize your soap recipes to healthy distinctive skin sorts and conditions, adding specific herbs and vital oils acknowledged for his or her healing houses.

ENVIRONMENTAL BENEFITS

Making your own soap is an remarkable way to reduce your environmental footprint. Commercial soaps regularly are available plastic packaging and include substances derived from unsustainable sources. Homemade cleaning soap making promotes eco-friendly practices that advantage the planet.

- Eco Friendly Ingredients: Use organic and sustainably sourced components that are biodegradable and mild at the environment.

- Reduced Waste: By developing your own soap, you may remove unnecessary packaging and reduce plastic waste.

Many cleaning soap makers use reusable molds and gear, further minimizing environmental effect.

ECONOMIC BENEFITS

Homemade cleaning soap may be a value effective opportunity to high give up industrial soaps.

- Cost Savings: Ingredients sold in bulk for cleaning soap making can result in huge savings over time. Plus, you can make big batches that last longer.

- Potential Income: Once you grow to be talented in soap making, you would possibly even don't forget selling your creations at local markets or on line, turning your interest right into a source of earnings.

CHAPTER 1: UNDERSTANDING SOAP AND ITS INGREDIENTS

WHAT IS SOAP?

EXPLANATION OF THE SOAP MAKING TECHNIQUE (SAPONIFICATION).

At the coronary heart of soap making lies a captivating chemical process referred to as saponification. Understanding this technique is prime to studying the artwork of cleaning soap making, making sure that every batch of soap you create is powerful, secure, and enjoyable to use.

WHAT IS SAPONIFICATION?

Saponification is the chemical response that happens when fats or oils come into touch with a sturdy alkali, usually sodium hydroxide (lye). This reaction transforms the fats and oils into soap and glycerin. Here's a simple breakdown of the procedure:

1. Fats and Oils: These are the main elements in cleaning soap making, imparting the fatty acids important for the response. Commonly used oils consist of olive oil, coconut oil, palm oil, and shea butter, every contributing extraordinary qualities to the final soap.

2. Alkali (Lye): Sodium hydroxide (for stable soap) or potassium hydroxide (for liquid soap) is the alkali used to cause saponification. When lye is mixed with water, it creates a fantastically alkaline answer that can react with fats and oils.

3. Water: Water acts as a medium to dissolve the lye and facilitate the saponification technique. It also helps in distributing the alkali frivolously for the duration of the oil mixture.

THE SAPONIFICATION PROCESS

The saponification method can be divided into several key steps:

1. Preparing the Lye Solution:

- Carefully measure the specified quantity of lye and water in step with your recipe.

- Slowly upload the lye to the water (in no way the opposite manner round) at the same time as stirring gently. This creates a tremendously exothermic response, meaning it will warmth up quick. Allow the lye approach to cool to the favored temperature.

2. Melting and Mixing Oils:

- Weigh and soften any stable oils (like coconut oil or shea butter) after which integrate them with liquid oils (like olive oil or sunflower oil) in a large bowl.

- Heat the oil combination gently till all oils are fully melted and well blended, then permit it to cool to the desired temperature, normally round one hundred and twenty°F (3849°C).

3. Combining Lye Solution and Oils:

- Once each the lye answer and the oils are at similar temperatures, slowly pour the lye solution into the oils.

- Use a stick blender to combinc the solution. This helps to emulsify the aggregate and hurries up the saponification technique.

4. Trace:

As you combo, the mixture will start to thicken. "Trace" is the point at which the cleaning soap combination thickens to a pudding like consistency. You can take a look at for hint by means of drizzling some of the soap combination on pinnacle of itself; if it leaves a seen path or "trace," it's ready.

5. Adding Additives:

- At hint, you may add important oils, colorants, and other components like herbs, clay, or exfoliants. Mix thoroughly to ensure even distribution.

6. Pouring into Molds:

- Pour the cleaning soap mixture into molds, smoothing the top with a spatula if important. Tap the molds lightly on the counter to launch any trapped air bubbles.

7. Curing:

- Cover the molds with a towel or blanket to insulate them and allow the saponification technique to complete. After 2448 hours, the cleaning soap may be unmolded and reduce into bars.

- The bars need to then be left to cure in a properly ventilated area for four6 weeks. This allows extra water to evaporate and the cleaning soap to harden, ensuing in a milder, longer lasting bar.

UNDERSTANDING THE CHEMISTRY

At the molecular level, saponification entails the hydrolysis of triglycerides (fat and oils) by means of the lye solution, breaking them down into glycerol (glycerin) and fatty acid salts (soap).

textFat (Triglyceride) textLye (NaOH) right arrow textGlycerin textSoap (Fatty Acid Salt)

The particular properties of the soap—including hardness, lather, and moisturizing ability—rely on the forms of fats and oils used, as every kind has a one of a kind fatty acid profile.

BASIC INGREDIENTS

Creating extraordinary herbal natural soap starts with know how the simple components concerned. Each aspect performs a essential position inside the cleaning soap making technique, influencing the properties, overall performance, and advantages of the very last product.

1. Oils and Fats

Oils and fats are the number one components in soap making, imparting the necessary fatty acids that react with lye to shape cleaning soap. Different oils contribute exclusive features to the soap, along with hardness, lather, and moisturizing properties.

- Olive Oil: Known for its moisturizing properties, olive oil produces a gentle soap with a creamy lather. It is good for touchy and dry skin.

- Coconut Oil: This oil creates a difficult bar with a rich, bubbly lather. However, an excessive amount of coconut oil may be drying, so it is regularly used in aggregate with different oils.

- Palm Oil: Palm oil contributes to the hardness and sturdiness of the cleaning soap. It produces a stable lather and is regularly used alongside other oils to balance the houses of the soap.

- Shea Butter: Rich in nutrients and fatty acids, shea butter provides moisturizing and conditioning qualities to cleaning soap. It is exquisite for creating a expensive, skin nourishing bar.

- Castor Oil: Known for its potential to reinforce lather, castor oil is regularly utilized in small amounts to decorate the bubble pleasant of cleaning soap.

- Sweet Almond Oil: This oil is lightweight and nourishing, presenting awesome moisturizing homes without leaving a greasy residue.

2. Lye (Sodium Hydroxide)

Lye, or sodium hydroxide, is a crucial factor in the saponification method. It is a notably caustic alkali that reacts with fats and oils to shape soap and glycerin. While lye itself is dangerous and ought to be treated with care, it's far completely converted at some stage in saponification, leaving no harmful residues in the completed soap.

- Safety Precautions: Always put on protective gear consisting of gloves, goggles, and lengthy sleeves whilst handling lye. Work in a nicely ventilated region and add lye to water (never the opposite manner round) to keep away from dangerous reactions.

3. Water

Water is used to dissolve the lye and facilitate the saponification procedure. It facilitates to distribute the lye flippantly all through the oil combination, making sure a whole and uniform response. The sort of water used can affect the satisfactory of the cleaning soap:

- Distilled Water: Distilled water is recommended for soap making as it's far free from impurities and minerals which could intrude with the saponification method.

- Herbal Teas and Infusions: For added advantages, you could use herbal teas or infusions in preference to undeniable water. These infusions can impart extra therapeutic homes and herbal shade to the soap.

4. Herbal Additives

Herbs and botanical components are what make herbal herbal soaps precise. They may be integrated in numerous bureaucracy, which includes dried herbs, herbal infusions, and essential oils, every contributing its very own set of benefits:

- Dried Herbs: Adding finely ground or entire dried herbs can offer exfoliation and natural shade. Common picks consist of lavender, chamomile, and calendula.

- Herbal Infusions: Steeping herbs in warm water or oil extracts their useful homes, which could then be delivered to the cleaning soap combination. For instance, an infusion of rosemary can decorate the soap's antiseptic features.

- Essential Oils: Essential oils are concentrated plant extracts that offer herbal perfume and healing advantages. Popular options encompass lavender, tea tree, peppermint, and eucalyptus oils.

5. Other Additives

In addition to the core ingredients, diverse other components can be blanketed to decorate the homes and aesthetics of your cleaning soap:

- Clay: Natural clay like kaolin, bentonite, and French green clay can offer coloration and extra cleaning homes.

- Exfoliants: Ingredients which includes oatmeal, floor coffee, and poppy seeds can add a mild exfoliating effect.

- Colorants: Natural colorants like turmeric, spirulina, and activated charcoal can be used to achieve vibrant, beautiful colorations.

OILS AND FATS: TYPES AND PROPERTIES

Oils and fat are the foundational substances in soap making, presenting the fatty acids vital for saponification and determining the very last features of the cleaning soap. Each form of oil or fat brings its precise properties, affecting hardness, lather, conditioning, and cleansing capability.

1. Olive Oil

- Properties: Moisturizing, mild, and conditioning.
- Benefits: Produces a slight soap with a creamy lather, appropriate for sensitive and dry skin.
- Usage: Often used as a big part of the oil blend. Pure Castile cleaning soap is made with one hundred% olive oil.
- Saponification Value (SAP): 0.134 (quantity of lye wished consistent with gram of oil).

2. Coconut Oil

Properties: Cleansing, hardening, and bubbly lather.

Benefits: Creates a tough bar of cleaning soap with a wealthy, fluffy lather. It has top notch cleansing properties.

Usage: Typically used at 2030% of the entire oil weight to avoid over drying the pores and skin.

SAP: 0.183.

3. Palm Oil

- Properties: Hardening, solid lather, and conditioning.
- Benefits: Adds hardness and longevity to soap, growing a balanced bar with strong lather.
- Usage: Often used at 2030% of the overall oil weight. Sustainable and ethically sourced palm oil ought to be used.

SAP: 0.141.

4. Shea Butter

- Properties: Moisturizing, conditioning, and creamy lather.
- Benefits: Adds luxurious moisturizing properties and is rich in nutrients A and E.
- Usage: Used at five15% of the full oil weight to beautify conditioning and creaminess.

SAP: 0.128.

5. Castor Oil

- Properties: Humectant, conditioning, and boosts lather.

- Benefits: Enhances the bubbly and creamy lather of the cleaning soap. It is likewise a tremendous moisturizer.

- Usage: Typically used at 510% of the total oil weight.

SAP: zero.128.

.6. Sweet Almond Oil

Properties: Light, conditioning, and moisturizing.

Benefits: Provides a soothing, moisturizing high quality, making it remarkable for touchy pores and skin.

Usage: Used at five10% of the full oil weight for added conditioning.

SAP: 0.136.

7. Avocado Oil

Properties: Rich, conditioning, and moisturizing.

Benefits: High in vitamins and fatty acids, it deeply nourishes and conditions the skin.

Usage: Used at 515% of the total oil weight.

SAP: 0.133.

8. Cocoa Butter

Properties: Hardening, conditioning, and creamy lather.

Benefits: Adds hardness and a wealthy, creamy lather. It is distinctly moisturizing and helps stabilize the cleaning soap.

Usage: Used at 515% of the overall oil weight.

SAP: zero.137.

9. Sunflower Oil

Properties: Light, conditioning, and moisturizing.

- Benefits: High in diet E and critical fatty acids, it is amazing for conditioning and moisturizing the skin.
- Usage: Used at 1020% of the overall oil weight.

SAP: zero.136.

LYE (SODIUM HYDROXIDE): SAFETY AND HANDLING

Lye, or sodium hydroxide (NaOH), is a crucial component in soap making, allowing the saponification process that transforms fat and oils into soap. While it's far a effective and integral component, it's also especially caustic and calls for cautious dealing with to make certain safety.

UNDERSTANDING LYE

- Chemical Nature: Lye is a sturdy alkali which could reason severe chemical burns and accidents if it comes into contact with the pores and skin, eyes, or breathing gadget.

- Importance in Soap Making: During saponification, lye reacts with fat and oils to create cleaning soap and glycerin. When well used and dealt with, no lye stays in the completed soap, making it secure for use.

SAFETY EQUIPMENT AND PRECAUTIONS

To safely deal with lye, it's miles essential to use the right shielding device and follow strict safety protocols:

1. Protective Gear:

- Gloves: Wear heavy obligation rubber or nitrite gloves to protect your palms from lye burns.

- Goggles: Use safety goggles to guard your eyes from splashes.

- Long Sleeves and Pants: Wear long sleeves, pants, and closed toe footwear to defend your skin from accidental splashes.

- Apron: A water resistant apron affords extra safety for your garb and frame.

2. Work Area:

- Ventilation: Work in a well ventilated region to avoid inhaling fumes. Using a fume hood or working outdoors is ideal.

- Clean and Clutter Free: Keep your work area smooth and freed from litter to prevent injuries.

3. Handling and Mixing Lye:

- Measuring: Accurately measure lye the usage of a virtual scale to make sure the appropriate ratio on your cleaning soap recipe.

- Mixing: Always add lye to water, by no means water to lye, to prevent a violent reaction that could motive splattering. Stir slowly and regularly.

Temperature: Be conscious that mixing lye with water generates warmness. Use a warmness resistant field to avoid cracking or breaking.

 Step by Step Lye Handling Process

1. Preparing the Lye Solution:

- Weigh the Lye: Using a digital scale, cautiously weigh the desired quantity of lye as in step with your soap recipe.

- Weigh the Water: Measure the specified quantity of water. It is crucial to use distilled water to avoid impurities that can affect the response.

- Add Lye to Water: Slowly pour the lye into the water while stirring constantly. Do this in a nicely ventilated location or under a fume hood to avoid breathing in the fumes.

- Stirring: Stir the answer until the lye is absolutely dissolved. The combination becomes hot, so handle it with care.

2. Cooling and Storing the Lye Solution:

- Cooling: Allow the lye technique to cool to the desired temperature, usually between one hundred twenty°F (38forty nine°C), earlier than mixing it with oils.

- Storage: If you want to save the lye solution, ensure it is in a genuinely classified, tightly sealed, and chemical resistant container. Keep it out of attain of children and pets.

EMERGENCY PROCEDURES

Despite taking precautions, injuries can happen. It's important to be organized:

1. Skin Contact:

- Rinse Immediately: If lye comes into contact with your pores and skin, rinse the affected region with copious quantities of bloodless water for at the least 15 mins. Do no longer use vinegar or every other neutralizing agent.

- Seek Medical Attention: If a burn develops or the affected location is huge, are seeking for scientific interest straight away.

2. Eye Contact:

- Flush with Water: If lye receives into your eyes, right now flush them with cold water for at least 15 mins and are looking for emergency scientific attention.

3. Inhalation:

- Fresh Air: If you inhale lye fumes, flow to an area with fresh air without delay. Seek medical interest if you revel in problem respiratory.

4. Ingestion:

- Do Not Induce Vomiting: If lye is ingested, do now not induce vomiting. Rinse the mouth thoroughly with water and seek instant medical interest.

WATER AND OTHER BEVERAGES (E.G., HERBAL TEAS, MILK).

Water and Other Liquids in Soap Making

Water is a crucial component in cleaning soap making, used to dissolve the lye and facilitate the saponification process. However, creative cleaning soap makers often alternative element or all the water with other beverages, including herbal teas, milk, or maybe fruit juices, to impart extra houses and advantages to the cleaning soap.

1. Water

- Distilled Water: The maximum common and recommended liquid for cleaning soap making. Distilled water is loose from impurities and minerals that may interfere with the saponification technique, ensuring a consistent and reliable final results.

- Benefits: Using distilled water allows hold the purity of your cleaning soap and stops undesirable reactions which can occur with tap water, along with discoloration or choppy texture.

2. Herbal Teas and Infusions

Herbal Teas: Herbal teas are made with the aid of steeping herbs in hot water. Popular alternatives encompass chamomile, lavender, peppermint, and rosemary. These teas can add healing properties and natural coloring to the soap.

- Preparation: Brew a strong tea by using extra herbs than you would for ingesting, then stress and funky the tea before mixing it with the lye. Remember that the lye will darken the shade of the tea.

- Benefits: Herbal teas can enhance the cleaning soap with natural scents and pores and skin advantages, inclusive of soothing or anti inflammatory homes from chamomile or antibacterial houses from rosemary.

3. Milk

- Types of Milk: Goat milk, cow milk, coconut milk, almond milk, and buttermilk are usually used in cleaning soap making. Goat milk is in particular popular because of its high fat content material and skin nourishing houses.

- Preparation: Milk needs to be frozen earlier than mixing with lye to save you sizzling and curdling. Slowly add lye to the frozen milk, stirring continuously to maintain the temperature low and save you the milk from burning.

- Benefits: Milk provides creaminess, a rich lather, and moisturizing characteristics to the soap. It is also wealthy in vitamins and proteins that nourish the skin.

4. Fruit and Vegetable Juices

● Juices: Freshly squeezed or pureed fruit and vegetable juices, inclusive of carrot, cucumber, apple, or orange juice, can be used. These juices add herbal color and vitamins to the soap.

● Preparation: Like milk, juices need to be frozen before blending with lye to prevent overheating and capacity sizzling. Juices also can introduce sugars, that may boost up the saponification manner and require cautious temperature manipulate.

● Benefits: Juices can offer vitamins, antioxidants, and a variety of natural hues. For example, carrot juice provides a vibrant orange coloration and is rich in beta carotene.

5. Beer and Wine

- Alcoholic Beverages: Beer and wine can be used to feature unique homes to cleaning soap. The sugars in these liquids can boom lather and contribute to a smoother texture.

- Preparation: Allow beer or wine to move flat through leaving it out for twentyfour48 hours to release the carbonation. Freeze the liquid before including lye to prevent a speedy reaction and capability spillage.

- Benefits: Beer consists of hops, that may soothe and melt the skin, while wine is rich in antioxidants.

HERBAL ADDITIVES

Herbal components are an incredible way to enhance the features and enchantment of herbal soaps. They deliver a variety of blessings, which include natural shade, exfoliation, and therapeutic houses.

TYPES OF HERBAL ADDITIVES

1. Dried Herbs

- Lavender: Known for its soothing and calming houses. Lavender can be delivered as complete buds or floor.

- Chamomile: Has anti inflammatory and calming results, making it perfect for touchy pores and skin. Use as dried plants or floor powder.

- Calendula: Offers recuperation and anti inflammatory houses. Use whole petals or infused in oil.

- Rose Petals: Provides mild exfoliation and a pleasing scent. Use dried and crushed.

- Peppermint: Adds a clean scent and cooling sensation. Use dried leaves or powder.

2. Herbal Infusions and Teas

- Preparation: Make a strong tea or infusion by means of steeping herbs in boiling water. Strain and cool before adding to the lye answer.

Examples:

- Rosemary: Known for its antiseptic homes and invigorating fragrance.

- Green Tea: Rich in antioxidants, inexperienced tea can assist to shield the pores and skin and add a gentle inexperienced hue.

3. Herbal Powders

- Turmeric: Adds a warm, golden coloration and has anti inflammatory houses.

- Spirulina: Provides a natural inexperienced color and is rich in vitamins and minerals.

- Activated Charcoal: Adds detoxifying homes and a striking black coloration.

4. Essential Oils

- Lavender Oil: Calming and soothing, perfect for all skin kinds.

- Tea Tree Oil: Antibacterial and anti fungal, properly for pimples inclined pores and skin.

- Eucalyptus Oil: Refreshing and antiseptic, first rate for invigorating the skin.

- Peppermint Oil: Provides a cooling sensation and a sparkling heady scent.

- Rosemary Oil: Stimulating and antiseptic, true for selling stream.

5. Herbal Clays

- Kaolin Clay: Gentle and appropriate for all skin sorts, provides mild exfoliation.

- French Green Clay: Known for its powerful detoxifying residences.

- Bentonite Clay: Adds a silky experience and is superb for oily skin types.

INCORPORATING HERBAL ADDITIVES

1. Timing: Add herbal additives at "hint," the point in cleaning soap making while the combination has thickened to a pudding like consistency. This ensures even distribution and preserves the houses of the herbs.

2. Amount: The quantity of natural additives depends on the type and favored impact. Start with small amounts (12 tablespoons in line with pound of oils) and regulate based on private desire and experimentation.

3. Preparation:

- Grinding: Finely grind herbs and flora the use of a coffee grinder or mortar and pestle to save you scratchiness and ensure even distribution.

- Infusing: Create natural infusions with the aid of steeping herbs in oil or water, then straining out the solids. Use the infused liquid in region of water or a part of the oil in your recipe.

- Blending: Mix powders and clays very well to save you clumping.

4. Examples of Herbal Soap Recipes:

- Lavender and Chamomile Soap: Combine dried lavender buds, chamomile vegetation, and lavender crucial oil for a relaxing and soothing soap.

- Green Tea and Lemongrass Soap: Use a sturdy inexperienced tea infusion and add lemongrass critical oil for an antioxidant rich and fresh soap.

- Turmeric and Honey Soap: Blend turmeric powder and honey for a moisturizing and anti inflammatory bar.

- Peppermint and Charcoal Soap: Combine activated charcoal and peppermint essential oil for a detoxifying and invigorating cleaning soap.

BENEFITS OF THE USAGE OF HERBS IN CLEANING SOAP.

Benefits of Using Herbs in Soap

Incorporating herbs into cleaning soap making can transform a simple bar of soap into a high priced, therapeutic product with a wide range of benefits. Herbs provide herbal scents, hues, and healing homes that beautify the overall great and attraction of self made cleaning soap.

1. Natural Fragrance

- Aromatherapy: Herbs offer a herbal and mild perfume which could have aroma therapeutic effects. For instance, lavender has calming residences, at the same time as peppermint is invigorating.

- Chemical Free: Unlike synthetic fragrances, herbal scents are unfastened from harmful chemical compounds and are much less in all likelihood to motive hypersensitive reactions.

2. Skin Benefits

- Anti Inflammatory: Herbs like chamomile and calendula have anti inflammatory houses, making them perfect for soothing angry or touchy pores and skin.

- Antibacterial and Anti fungal: Herbs along with tea tree, rosemary, and thyme own antibacterial and anti fungal residences, which can help in treating acne and other skin conditions.

- Moisturizing: Herbs like aloe vera and calendula help in retaining moisture and retaining the pores and skin hydrated.

- Healing: Herbs like comfrey and calendula promote wound recuperation and may be beneficial for minor cuts and abrasions.

3. Natural Colorants

- Vibrant Colors: Herbs can provide a wide variety of herbal coloring to soap, from the deep inexperienced of spirulina to the golden yellow of turmeric.

- No Synthetic Dyes: Using herbs as colorants avoids the need for synthetic dyes, which can be harsh at the pores and skin and are regularly derived from petrochemicals.

4. Exfoliation

- Gentle Exfoliates: Ground herbs, seeds, and plants can act as mild exfoliants, helping to get rid of useless skin cells and sell a wholesome glow. Examples encompass floor oatmeal, lavender buds, and poppy seeds.

- Improved Texture: The inclusion of exfoliating herbs can improve the feel and experience of the soap, offering a moderate scrubbing movement.

5. Antioxidant Properties

- Skin Protection: Many herbs are wealthy in antioxidants, that may protect the skin from free radicals and environmental damage. Green tea and rosemary are awesome examples.

- Anti Aging: Antioxidants in herbs can help in reducing the symptoms of growing older via promoting collagen manufacturing and enhancing pores and skin elasticity.

6. Therapeutic Properties

- Calming and Relaxing: Herbs like lavender, chamomile, and valerian root have calming and relaxing properties, that could help lessen strain and improve sleep nice.

CHAPTER 2: ESSENTIAL TOOLS AND EQUIPMENT

LIST OF NECESSARY TOOLS

MIXING BOWLS, THERMOMETERS, MOLDS, SCALES, AND SO ON.

Certainly, having the proper device and gear is crucial for a success cleaning soap making.

Equipment for Soap Making:

1. Mixing Bowls:

- Stainless Steel or Heat Resistant Plastic: Use nonreactive blending bowls that can resist warmness whilst running with lye.

2. Thermometer:

- Digital Thermometer: Essential for monitoring the temperature of oils and lye strategy to ensure they're in the desired range for saponification.

3. Molds:

●   Silicone Molds: Ideal for novices as they are bendy and clean to unmold. Choose molds of various sizes and styles according to your alternatives.

●   Wooden or Plastic Molds: Can be used for larger batches and conventional bar shapes.

4. Scales:

●   Digital Scale: Accurate size of ingredients with the aid of weight is critical for consistency and the success of your soap batches.

5. Stick Blender or Hand Mixer:

●   Stick Blender: Preferred for soap making as it emulsifies the oils and lye solution quick, speeding up the saponification manner.

●   Hand Mixer: Can be used as an alternative if a stick blender is not available, but may additionally take longer to reach trace.

6. Protective Gear:

- Gloves: Heavy obligation rubber or nitrile gloves to shield your fingers from lye.

- Goggles: Safety goggles to shield your eyes from splashes.

- Apron: Waterproof apron to shield your garb.

7. Lye Safe Containers:

- Heat Resistant Containers: Use glass or stainless steel containers for blending lye and water. Avoid aluminum or reactive materials.

8. Stirring Utensils:

Stainless Steel Spoons or Whisks: Nonreactive utensils for mixing oils, lye answer, and components.

9. Safety Equipment:

- Ventilation: Work in a nicely ventilated vicinity or use a fume hood to deplete lye fumes.

- First Aid Kit: Have a first useful resource kit available in case of sweet sixteen injuries or spills.

- Emergency Contacts: Keep emergency touch numbers quite simply reachable.

10. Miscellaneous:

- Parchment Paper or Freezer Paper: Line molds with parchment or freezer paper for smooth cleaning soap removal.

- Plastic Wrap or Towels: Use plastic wrap or towels to cover molds in the course of the curing method.

- Labels and Markers: Label cleaning soap batches with substances, date of creating, and curing time.

TIPS FOR EQUIPMENT CARE AND SAFETY:

1. Cleanliness: Ensure all gadget and utensils are clean and loose from contaminants earlier than use to keep away from affecting the best of your cleaning soap.

2. Storage: Store lye and other chemical substances in a fab, dry location, away from moisture and direct daylight. Keep out of attain of children and pets.

3. Maintenance: Regularly smooth and hold your gadget to extend their lifespan and save you cross infection.

4. Safety First: Always prioritize safety whilst coping with lye and other chemicals. Wear protecting tools, work in a properly ventilated area, and comply with safety tips rigorously.

SAFETY EQUIPMENT

Safety system is crucial when running with potentially risky substances like lye in cleaning soap making.

1. Protective Clothing:

1. Gloves:

- Material: Heavy obligation, chemical resistant gloves product of rubber or nitrile.

- Purpose: Protect your arms from direct contact with lye and chemical compounds, stopping burns and irritation.

2. Eye Protection:

Safety Goggles:

Type: Wraparound fashion goggles for entire eye protection.

Purpose: Shield your eyes from splashes of lye or soap combination, stopping eye inflammation and damage.

3. Clothing:

Long Sleeved Shirt and Pants:

Material: Wear garb product of herbal fibers like cotton, as they are much less probable to soften or catch fire in case of unintentional splashes.

Purpose: Cover your pores and skin to decrease publicity to lye and chemicals.

4. Apron:

Waterproof Apron:

Material: Choose an apron made from water resistant fabric to protect your apparel.

Purpose: Prevent spills and splashes from reaching your clothes, ensuring your protection and maintaining your apparel.

2. Respiratory Protection:

1. Ventilation:

Well Ventilated Area:

Location: Work in a nicely ventilated room or set up a fume hood for proper air circulate.

Purpose: Reduce inhalation of fumes from lye and chemicals, promoting a more secure running surroundings.

2. Masks:

Respirator Mask:

Type: N95 or P100 respirator mask with appropriate filters for chemical fumes.

Purpose: Protect your lungs from breathing in harmful vapors and fumes generated at some stage in cleaning soap making.

3. First Aid Kit:

1. Basic First Aid Supplies:

Bandages: Assorted adhesive bandages for minor cuts and abrasions.

Antiseptic Wipes/Solution: Antiseptic wipes or option to smooth wounds and prevent infections.

Burn Cream/Gel: Burn cream or gel for treating minor burns as a result of lye or warm soap mixture.

Gauze Pads: Sterile gauze pads for protecting larger wounds or burns.

Tweezers and Scissors: Tweezers for putting off splinters and scissors for cutting bandages or gauze.

GLOVES, GOGGLES, APRONS, AND PROPER AIR FLOW.

Absolutely, having the proper private defensive gadget (PPE) and making sure proper air flow are essential protection measures when working with lye and different chemical substances in soap making.

1. Gloves:

- Material: Choose heavy obligation gloves manufactured from rubber or nitrile, as they provide top chemical resistance.

- Fit: Ensure the gloves suit snugly however readily to save you them from slipping off during work.

Function: Protect your hands from direct touch with lye and chemicals, stopping burns and irritation.

2. Goggles:

Type: Opt for safety goggles that provide a good seal round your eyes, which include wraparound styles.

Clear Vision: Ensure the goggles do no longer obstruct your imaginative and prescient and will let you see actually while running.

Function: Shield your eyes from splashes of lye or soap mixture, preventing eye inflammation and injury.

3. Aprons:

Material: Use a water resistant apron fabricated from durable material to guard your clothing correctly.

Coverage: Choose an apron that covers your torso and lower body to save you spills and splashes from achieving your clothes.

Function: Protect your apparel from stains and chemical publicity, ensuring your protection and keeping your apparel.

4. Proper Ventilation:

- Location: Work in a well ventilated area, along with near an open window or use a fume hood if available.

- Air Circulation: Ensure there may be good enough air stream to disperse any fumes or vapors generated during cleaning soap making.

- Purpose: Reduce inhalation of potentially harmful fumes and create a safer working environment for your self.

CREATING A SAFE AND EFFICIENT WORKSPACE.

Creating a safe and efficient workspace for cleaning soap making entails several key steps to make certain your safety, the best of your products, and an fun crafting experience.

1. Choose the Right Location:

Ventilation: Select a properly ventilated place to disperse fumes and prevent inhaling doubtlessly harmful vapors. Consider operating close to a window, the usage of a fan, or putting in a fume hood if to be had.

Dedicated Space: Designate a specific place for soap making to avoid cross contamination with meals or other household items.

Accessibility: Ensure your workspace is without problems reachable and well lit to facilitate clean workflow and visibility.

2. Organize Your Tools and Supplies:

Storage: Keep your cleaning soap making substances, including oils, lye, molds, and equipment, organized and easily on hand. Use shelves, shelves, or storage packing containers to keep order.

Labeling: Clearly label all bins and bottles to perceive elements and keep away from confusion.

Spill Containment: Have spill kits or absorbent substances on hand to fast easy up any spills or accidents.

3. Personal Protective Equipment (PPE):

Gloves: Wear chemical resistant gloves made from rubber or nitrile to defend your palms from lye and other chemical substances.

Goggles: Use protection goggles or glasses with side shields to guard your eyes from splashes and fumes.

Apron: Wear a water resistant apron to defend your garb from spills and splashes.

4. Equipment and Tools:

Mixing Bowls and Utensils: Use nonreactive materials including stainless steel or warmness resistant plastic for mixing oils, lye, and components.

Thermometer: Have a digital thermometer to monitor temperatures as it should be all through the soap making method.

Stick Blender or Hand Mixer: Use a stick blender for emulsifying the soap combination quick and efficiently.

Molds: Choose molds made of silicone, timber, or plastic which can be suitable for cleaning soap making and easy to unmold.

5. Safety Procedures:

Read Instructions: Familiarize yourself with the producer's instructions for coping with lye, oils, and different chemical substances. Follow cleaning soap recipes cautiously.

Work Methodically: Follow a step by means of step technique and keep away from speeding via the procedure to decrease injuries.

Emergency Preparedness: Keep a primary useful resource kit, emergency contact numbers, and a hearth extinguisher nearby.

CHAPTER 3: THE BASICS OF SOAP MAKING

TYPES OF SOAP MAKING PROCESSES

COLD SYSTEM.

Cold process soap making is a conventional approach that entails growing soap from scratch the use of oils, lye (sodium hydroxide), and water.

Ingredients Needed:

1. Oils and Fats:

Choose a mixture of oils including olive oil, coconut oil, palm oil, shea butter, cocoa butter, and others based totally on the properties you want on your soap (hardness, lather, conditioning, and so forth.).

2. Lye (Sodium Hydroxide):

Essential for saponification, the chemical response that turns oils into cleaning soap.

Ensure to deal with lye with caution and use right safety gear.

3. Water:

Distilled water is suggested to keep away from impurities that may affect the soap's pleasant.

4. Additives (Optional):

Herbs, crucial oils, colorants, exfoliants, and other additives for fragrance, color, and extra benefits.

Equipment Needed:

1. Safety Gear:

Gloves, goggles, and an apron to defend your self from lye and other chemical substances.

2. Mixing Equipment:

Heat resistant boxes for blending oils and lye answer.

Stainless metallic or plastic mixing spoons or whisks.

3. Thermometer:

Digital thermometer to monitor temperatures appropriately.

4. Stick Blender:

Used for emulsifying the oils and lye answer fast.

5. Soap Molds:

Silicone molds, wooden molds, or plastic molds for shaping and curing the soap.

6. Workspace:

Well ventilated region with right lights and get entry to to water and cleansing elements.

HOT PROCEDURE.

Hot manner soap making is a version of soap making that entails heating the soap aggregate after saponification has passed off. This technique hurries up the saponification method, making the soap geared up to apply extra quick than cold process soap.

INGREDIENTS NEEDED:

1. Oils and Fats:

Use a mix of oils which includes olive oil, coconut oil, palm oil, shea butter, cocoa butter, and so on., based in your preferred soap residences.

2. Lye (Sodium Hydroxide):

Essential for saponification, the chemical response that turns oils into soap. Handle lye with warning and use proper safety equipment.

3. Water:

Distilled water is usually recommended to keep away from impurities which could have an effect on soap fine.

4. Additives (Optional):

Herbs, important oils, colorants, exfoliants, and different additives for perfume, colour, and extra blessings.

EQUIPMENT NEEDED:

1. Safety Gear:

Gloves, goggles, and an apron to protect yourself from lye and other chemicals.

2. Mixing Equipment:

Heat resistant boxes for blending oils and lye answer.

Stainless steel or plastic mixing spoons or whisks.

3. Thermometer:

Digital thermometer to display temperatures accurately.

4. Stick Blender (Optional):

Used for emulsifying the oils and lye answer if wanted.

5. Crock pot or Slow Cooker:

Used for heating and cooking the cleaning soap combination.

Step via Step Guide to Cold Process Soap Making

Step 1: Safety Precautions

1. Wear Protective Gear: Put on gloves, safety goggles, and an apron to guard your

self from lye and different chemical substances.

2. Work in a Well Ventilated Area: Ensure true airflow to keep away from breathing in fumes.

Step 2: Gather Ingredients and Equipment

1. Ingredients:

Oils and fats (e.G., olive oil, coconut oil, palm oil, shea butter)

Lye (sodium hydroxide)

Distilled water

Optional additives (vital oils, herbs, colorants)

2. Equipment:

Heat resistant boxes for blending

Digital scale for accurate measurements

Thermometer

Stick blender or hand mixer

Soap molds

Step 3: Prepare Lye Solution

1. Measure Ingredients: Weigh the desired quantity of lye and distilled water one after the other the usage of the virtual scale.

2. Mix Lye and Water: Slowly add lye to water in a heat resistant field, stirring gently until absolutely dissolved. Never upload water to lye.

3. Cool Lye Solution: Allow the lye technique to cool to round a hundreda hundred and twenty°F (3849°C) while stirring every now and then.

Step 4: Prepare Oils

1. Measure Oils: Weigh the oils and fat consistent with your soap recipe the usage of the digital scale.

2. Melt Solid Oils: If the use of solid oils like coconut oil or shea butter, melt them lightly on low heat until liquid.

Step 5: Mix Lye Solution and Oils

1. Check Temperatures: Ensure both the lye answer and oils are inside a comparable

temperature range, ideally around 100120°F (3849°C).

2. Combine: Pour the lye solution into the oils, using a spatula to scrape any remaining lye or oils from the boxes.

3. Blend: Use a stick blender or hand mixer to combo the aggregate till it reaches "hint," akin to thin pudding or custard. This indicates the beginning of saponification.

DETAILED INSTRUCTIONS WITH PHOTOS/ILLUSTRATIONS.

I can manual you through the procedure little by little, but I cannot provide photos or illustrations at once. However, you may easily discover particular tutorials with visible aids online.

Step 1: Safety Precautions

1. Wear Protective Gear: Put on gloves, safety goggles, and an apron to protect your self.

2. Work in a Well Ventilated Area: Ensure desirable airflow to avoid inhaling fumes.

 Step 2: Gather Ingredients and Equipment

1. Ingredients:

Oils and fat (e.G., olive oil, coconut oil, palm oil, shea butter)

Lye (sodium hydroxide)

Distilled water

Optional additives (crucial oils, herbs, colorants)

2. Equipment:

Heat resistant packing containers for mixing

Digital scale for accurate measurements

Thermometer

Stick blender or hand mixer

Soap molds

 Step 3: Prepare Lye Solution

1. Measure Ingredients: Weigh the lye and distilled water one after the other.

2. Mix Lye and Water: Slowly add lye to water in a warm resistant box, stirring till absolutely dissolved. Allow it to cool.

Step 4: Prepare Oils

1. Measure Oils: Weigh the oils and fat in keeping with your recipe.

2. Melt Solid Oils: If using stable oils, soften them lightly until liquid.

Step 5: Mix Lye Solution and Oils

1. Check Temperatures: Ensure each the lye solution and oils are round one hundred120°F (38forty nine°C).

2. Combine: Pour the lye solution into the oils.

3. Blend: Use a stick blender or hand mixer till the combination reaches "hint."

Step 6: Add Additives (Optional)

1. Essential Oils: Add for fragrance.

2. Herbs or Colorants: Add as favored.

MELT AND POUR SOAP MAKING

Melt and pour soap making is a amateur pleasant approach that entails melting premade soap bases, adding colorants, fragrances, and different additives, then pouring the mixture into molds to set.

Step 1: Gather Materials

1. Soap Base:

- Choose a soften and pour cleaning soap base, together with glycerin, shea butter, goat's milk, or coconut oil base.

2. Colorants:

Soap dyes, micas, or natural colorants like turmeric, spirulina, or cocoa powder.

3. Fragrances:

Essential oils, perfume oils, or herbs for scent.

4. Additives (Optional):

Exfoliants (e.G., oatmeal, espresso grounds), botanical (e.G., lavender buds), or other components for texture and appearance.

5. Molds:

Silicone molds, plastic molds, or cleaning soap loaf molds.

6. Equipment:

Micro wave safe field or double boiler for melting.

Stirring utensil (spoon or spatula).

Spray bottle with rubbing alcohol (for eliminating air bubbles).

Thermometer (elective).

Step 2: Prepare Workspace and Tools

1. Cleanliness:

Ensure your workspace and tools are easy and dry.

2. Organize Ingredients:

Arrange all substances and equipment inside smooth reach.

CHAPTER 4: INCORPORATING HERBS INTO YOUR SOAP

PREPARING HERBS FOR SOAP MAKING

DRYING AND STORING HERBS.

Drying and storing herbs properly is crucial to preserve their flavor, aroma, and medicinal properties.

Step 1: Harvesting Herbs

1. Timing: Harvest herbs inside the morning after the dew has dried however before the solar gets too hot. This is when the oils are most concentrated.

2. Method: Use smooth and sharp scissors or shears to reduce herbs. Harvest most effective wholesome and pest free components of the plant.

3. Leave Growth: Leave sufficient boom on the plant for it to preserve developing and thriving.

Step 2: Cleaning Herbs

1. Rinse: Gently rinse harvested herbs under cold water to get rid of dust, insects, and debris.

2. Pat Dry: Use a smooth material or paper towels to pat the herbs dry. Remove extra moisture to save you mildew throughout the drying procedure.

Step 3: Drying Methods

1. Air Drying:

- Bundle Herbs: Tie herbs into small bundles the usage of string or rubber bands. Keep the bundles small to make sure right airflow.

- Hanging: Hang the herb bundles the other way up in a heat, dry, and nicely ventilated vicinity out of direct daylight. Use a dark ish place to maintain colour.

- Drying Time: Depending on humidity and herb kind, it could take 12 weeks for herbs to dry absolutely.

2. Oven Drying (for brief drying):

- Spread Herbs: Arrange clean and dry herbs in a single layer on a baking sheet lined with parchment paper.

- Oven Temperature: Set the oven to the lowest temperature (generally round 140a hundred and fifty°F or 6065°C).

Drying Time: Check herbs frequently. It can also take 1four hours for herbs to dry very well.

3. Dehydrator (for regular drying):

Follow the manufacturer's commands on your dehydrator version.

Set the dehydrator to the perfect temperature for herbs (normally around ninety five one hundred fifteen°F or 35forty six°C).

Drying Time: Typically takes 14 hours, relying at the herb and dehydrator settings.

 Step 4: Storing Dried Herbs

1. Cooling: Allow dried herbs to chill completely before storing to save you condensation.

2. Storage Containers: Use hermetic glass jars, metallic tins, or resealable luggage to keep dried herbs.

3. Labeling: Label packing containers with the herb call and date of drying to music freshness.

4. Storage Conditions:

Location: Store dried herbs in a cool, darkish, and dry place away from direct sunlight, warmness, and moisture.

Avoid Humidity: Keep herbs away from the stove, dishwasher, or areas prone to humidity (like lavatories).

Shelf Life: Properly dried and saved herbs can last 6 months to one 12 months, however efficiency may additionally decrease through the years.

Making herbal infusions and teas. Making natural infusions and teas is a fantastic manner to revel in the flavors and healing benefits of herbs.

HERBAL INFUSIONS:

1. Choose Herbs:

Select clean or dried herbs based for your preferred flavor and advantages. Common herbs for infusions consist of chamomile, peppermint, lavender, lemon balm, and ginger.

2. Preparation:

Use 1 tablespoon of dried herbs or 2 tablespoons of fresh herbs consistent with cup of hot water.

Place the herbs in a teapot, glass jar, or mug.

3. Heat Water:

Heat water to simply below boiling (round one hundred eighty200°F or 82ninety three°C).

4. Pour Water:

Pour the hot water over the herbs within the teapot or mug.

5. Steep:

Cover the box to lure the steam and permit the herbs steep for 510 mins. Steeping time may additionally vary based totally at the herb and preferred energy.

6. Strain:

After steeping, stress the herbs the use of a great mesh sieve, tea strainer, or cheesecloth to get rid of solids.

7. Serve:

Pour the natural infusion into a cup and enjoy hot. You can add honey, lemon, or different sweeteners to flavor.

HERBAL TEAS:

1. Choose Herbs:

- Select herbs appropriate for brewing tea, which includes chamomile, green tea, hibiscus, rose hips, or rooibos.

2. Preparation:

- Use 1 teaspoon of dried herbs or 1 tablespoon of fresh herbs consistent with cup of warm water.

3. Heat Water:

Heat water to the suitable temperature based on the type of herb you're the use of. Different herbs might also require exceptional water temperatures (e.G., inexperienced tea at a hundred seventy five°F or 80°C).

4. Place Herbs:

Place the herbs in a teapot, infuser, or directly right into a mug.

5. Pour Water:

Pour the recent water over the herbs.

6. Steep:

- Cover the box and let the herbs steep for the recommended time (normally 35 mins for most natural teas).

7. Strain (if wished):

If the usage of unfastened herbs, pressure the tea the use of a tea strainer or infuser to get rid of solids.

8. Serve:

Pour the natural tea into a cup and revel in hot. Add sweeteners or flavorings if desired.

Adding Herbs to Soap

Adding herbs to soap can enhance its look, heady scent, or even upload beneficial houses.

Step 1: Choose Herbs

1. Select Herbs:

Choose dried herbs that complement the cleaning soap's fragrance or offer pores and skin blessings. Examples encompass lavender, chamomile, rosemary, calendula, peppermint, and rose petals.

2. Prepare Herbs:

Dry fresh herbs thoroughly to cast off moisture. You can air dry them or use a dehydrator.

Crush or grind dried herbs into smaller portions for less difficult incorporation into the soap.

 Step 2: Prepare Soap Base

1. Choose Soap Base:

Use a soften and pour soap base or make bloodless system cleaning soap from scratch. Ensure the bottom is suitable for including herbs.

If using a melt and pour base, soften it according to the manufacturer's commands.

2. Prepare Molds:

Prepare cleaning soap molds with the aid of lining them with parchment paper or silicone liners.

Step 3: Add Herbs

1. Timing:

If making soften and pour soap, upload herbs just earlier than pouring the melted cleaning soap into molds.

For bloodless method cleaning soap, add herbs at hint (when the cleaning soap has thickened however is still pourable).

2. Quantity:

Use 12 tablespoons of dried herbs in keeping with pound of soap base. Adjust the quantity based to your preference for herb concentration.

3. Incorporation:

Melt and Pour Soap: Sprinkle dried herbs into the melted cleaning soap base and stir gently to distribute frivolously.

Cold Process Soap: Add dried herbs to the cleaning soap mixture at trace and stir nicely to make sure even distribution.

Step 4: Pour and Cure Soap

1. Pour Soap Mixture:

Pour the soap mixture into prepared molds, making sure the herbs are calmly dispersed.

2. Curing:

For melt and pour cleaning soap, permit it to chill and harden absolutely within the molds.

For bloodless system soap, permit it to remedy in the molds for 46 weeks to harden and completely saponify.

Step 5: Unmold and Cut (for Cold Process Soap)

1. Unmold:

After curing, eliminate the soap from the molds.

For melt and pour cleaning soap, pass to the subsequent step after unmolding.

2. Cut:

Cut bloodless manner cleaning soap into bars the usage of a cleaning soap cutter or knife. Ensure the herbs are frivolously distributed at some stage in each bar.

Step 6: Label and Store

1. Label:

Label your herbal cleaning soap bars with the components used and the date of creating.

2. Store:

Store cleaning soap bars in a groovy, dry area faraway from moisture and direct sunlight.

Use within 612 months for nice best.

Tips for maintaining coloration and perfume.

Maintaining the colour and perfume of soap requires cautious managing, garage, and aspect selection.

For Color:

1. Choose Stable Colorants:

- Use colorants specifically designed for soap making, together with micas, oxide pigments, or natural colorants like clays and botanical powders.

Avoid the usage of water soluble dyes or food colors, as they'll fade or bleed over time.

2. Proper Mixing:

Ensure thorough blending of colorants into the soap base to obtain even color distribution.

Mix colorants into the cleaning soap aggregate at a slight temperature to prevent colorants from clumping or settling.

3. Avoid Overheating:

Avoid overheating the soap base in the course of melting or curing, as excessive temperatures can purpose colorants to vanish or trade.

Use a double boiler or microwave in brief bursts while melting cleaning soap base to control temperature.

4. Test Stability:

Test coloration balance by means of slicing a small piece of soap and exposing it to mild, warmness, and moisture. Monitor changes in coloration over time.

5. Protect from Light:

Store finished soap in opaque or dark coloured boxes to protect towards light exposure, that can fade shades.

FOR FRAGRANCE:

1. Use Quality Fragrances:

Use first rate fragrance oils or critical oils specifically formulated for soap making.

Ensure the perfume oils are pores and skin safe and do no longer include additives that could affect cleaning soap great.

2. Proper Scenting:

Add perfume oils or critical oils to the cleaning soap aggregate at the precise degree (e.G., during hint for cold procedure cleaning soap or whilst melting for soften and pour cleaning soap).

Use the advocated utilization charges provided by the perfume supplier to avoid overpowering scents or potential skin inflammation.

3. Stir Gently:

Stir fragrance oils or vital oils into the cleaning soap combination lightly but thoroughly to make certain even distribution without causing air bubbles.

4. Avoid Excessive Heat:

Minimize exposure to high temperatures at some stage in soap making and curing, as heat can reason fragrances to burn up greater fast.

Store soap in a fab, dry place faraway from warmth resources and direct daylight.

CHAPTER 5: CREATING YOUR OWN RECIPES

UNDERSTANDING OIL PROPERTIES

HARD VS. GENTLE OILS.

Hard oils and gentle oils are forms of oils used in soap making, each contributing precise homes to the completed cleaning soap.

Hard Oils:

1. Examples:

- Coconut oil
- Palm oil
- Cocoa butter
- Shea butter
- Mango butter

2. Characteristics:

- Solid at room temperature or have a excessive melting factor.
- Contribute hardness, balance, and lather to cleaning soap.

- Can be used as the primary base oils in soap recipes.
- High in saturated fatty acids, which provide cleansing homes.

3. Usage:

- Hard oils are utilized in cleaning soap making to create a corporation, long lasting bar of soap.
- They assist the soap bar maintain its form and sturdiness.
- Hard oils are frequently combined with smooth oils to balance cleaning and moisturizing homes.

Soft Oils:

1. Examples:

- Olive oil
- Sweet almond oil
- Avocado oil
- Sunflower oil
- Jojoba oil

2. Characteristics:

- Liquid at room temperature or have a low melting point.
- Contribute moisturizing, conditioning, and emollient residences to cleaning soap.
- Rich in unsaturated fatty acids, vitamins, and antioxidants.
- Provide a creamy lather and mild cleansing.

3. Usage:

- Soft oils are used in cleaning soap making to feature nourishing and moisturizing benefits.
- They assist balance the cleaning consequences of hard oils, making the cleaning soap gentle on the skin.
- Soft oils are regularly used in higher proportions in soap recipes for their conditioning properties.

CHOOSING OILS FOR SOAP MAKING:

1. Balance:

- A exact soap recipe typically includes a stability of hard and smooth oils to obtain preferred cleansing, lathering, and moisturizing residences.

- Adjust the ratio of tough and gentle oils primarily based on the form of cleaning soap you want to create (e.G., cleaning bars, moisturizing bars, forte bars).

2. Skin Type:

- Consider the pores and skin sort of intended users whilst selecting oils. For dry or touchy pores and skin, prioritize tender oils with high moisturizing properties. For oily or pimples susceptible skin, encompass difficult oils with cleaning homes.

3. Experiment:

- Experiment with exclusive combos of tough and smooth oils to create unique cleaning soap formulations.

- Keep a file of your recipes and word the homes of each oil to refine your cleaning soap making strategies.

FATTY ACID PROFILES AND THEIR EFFECTS ON SOAP.

The fatty acid profile of oils and fat used in soap making directly influences the houses of the ensuing soap, which include its cleaning capability, lather satisfactory, hardness, and conditioning houses.

Saturated Fatty Acids:

1. Lauric Acid:

Found in oils like coconut oil and palm kernel oil.

- Contributes to a difficult bar of soap with accurate lather and cleaning homes.

- Can be drying in high concentrations, so stability with other fatty acids for milder soap.

2. Mysticism Acid:

- Found in oils like coconut oil and palm kernel oil.
- Adds hardness and cleansing to cleaning soap.
- Can contribute to a fluffy lather but can be drying in excess.

3. Stearic Acid:

- Found in oils like cocoa butter and shea butter.
- Adds hardness and balance to cleaning soap bars.
- Creates a creamy lather and contributes to a moisturizing feel.
- Monounsaturated Fatty Acids:

1. Oleic Acid:

- Found in oils like olive oil, avocado oil, and sweet almond oil.

- Provides conditioning and moisturizing homes to soap.
- Produces a moderate, creamy lather and contributes to a softer bar.

POLYUNSATURATED FATTY ACIDS:

1. Linoleic Acid:

- Found in oils like sunflower oil, safflower oil, and grape seed oil.
- Adds conditioning and moisturizing houses to cleaning soap.
- Can contribute to a stable lather and a softer feel in cleaning soap.

2. Linolenic Acid:

- Found in oils like flax seed oil and hemp seed oil.
- Adds conditioning homes and might make contributions to a smoother texture in soap.

EFFECTS ON SOAP PROPERTIES:

1. Cleansing:

- Higher concentrations of lauric acid and myristic acid bring about a greater cleaning soap however may be drying if no longer balanced with conditioning oils.

- Balanced ratios of saturated, monounsaturated, and polyunsaturated fatty acids create a soap that cleanses efficaciously without stripping the skin.

FORMULATING YOUR OWN RECIPES

Formulating your own soap recipes allows you to personalize the houses of your soap consistent with your choices and desires.

Step 1: Understand Soap Making Basics

1. Know Your Ingredients:

- Learn about special oils, fat, lye (sodium hydroxide or potassium hydroxide), water, and additives used in cleaning soap making.

- Understand the residences of each ingredient, which include cleansing, conditioning, hardness, lather, and moisturizing results.

2. Learn About Fatty Acids:

- Familiarize yourself with the fatty acid profiles of oils and the way they affect soap properties.

- Balance the chances of saturated, monounsaturated, and polyunsaturated fatty acids for preferred soap characteristics.

3. Safety Precautions:

- Understand the safety measures required whilst working with lye, such as wearing protecting gear and dealing with lye answer cautiously.

Step 2: Set Your Soap Objectives

1. Define Soap Properties:

- Determine the favored traits of your cleaning soap, including cleaning capacity, lather type (creamy or bubbly), hardness, conditioning, and fragrance retention.

2. Consider Skin Types:

● Tailor your recipe to fit precise skin sorts (e.G., dry, sensitive, oily) or cope with skin worries (e.G., pimples, eczema).

Step 3: Choose Your Oils and Fats

1. Select Base Oils:

● Choose a combination of tough oils (e.G., coconut oil, palm oil, cocoa butter) and smooth oils (e.G., olive oil, candy almond oil, avocado oil).

● Consider the fatty acid profiles and properties of every oil to reap your soap objectives.

2. Calculate Percentages:

● Calculate the chances of each oil primarily based to your recipe's total oil weight. Use a soap calculator for accurate measurements and to make sure the recipe is lye balanced.

Step 4: Determine Lye and Water Amounts

1. Use a Soap Calculator:

- Input your preferred oils and their chances right into a soap calculator along side the desired super fat percent (normally five eight% for most recipes).

- The calculator will provide the right quantities of lye and water wanted for saponification.

Step 5: Add Additives and Fragrances

1. Select Additives:

- Decide on optionally available components which include critical oils, herbs, colorants, exfoliants, and different botanical.

- Consider their advantages, compatibility with the base oils, and preferred effects at the cleaning soap.

2. Calculate Additive Amounts:

● Calculate the percentages of additives based totally on the whole oil weight. Ensure to follow encouraged usage quotes for important oils and components.

Step 6: Test and Adjust

1. Make a Small Batch:

● Start with a small batch to check your recipe before making large quantities.

● Evaluate the cleaning soap's residences after curing, which includes lather, hardness, conditioning, fragrance, and skin sense.

2. Adjust as Needed:

Make adjustments to the recipe if the cleaning soap would not meet your expectancy. Modify oil percentages, super fat level, or additives as a result.

BALANCING CLEANING, MOISTURIZING, AND LATHERING PROPERTIES.

Balancing cleaning, moisturizing, and lathering residences is essential for developing a well rounded and powerful soap.

1. Choose Cleansing Oils:

- Include oils high in lauric acid and myristic acid for cleaning homes. Examples include coconut oil and palm kernel oil.

- Balance excessive cleaning oils with moisturizing oils to prevent the soap from being too drying.

2. Use Lye Concentration:

- Adjust the lye concentration in your cleaning soap recipe to govern the cleaning houses. Higher lye concentration will increase cleaning, at the same time as lower attention reduces it.

3. Consider Super fatting:

- Super fatting refers to leaving a percentage of unsaponified oils within the soap. A better super fat percentage consequences in a milder and much less stripping cleaning soap.

BALANCING MOISTURIZING:

1. Include Conditioning Oils:

- Incorporate oils excessive in oleic acid and other monounsaturated fatty acids for conditioning and moisturizing outcomes. Examples include olive oil, avocado oil, and candy almond oil.

- Use oils with high tiers of polyunsaturated fatty acids like linoleic acid for added moisturizing properties.

2. Adjust Super fat Level:

- Increase the super fat percentage to your recipe to enhance moisturizing residences. A better super fat level leaves greater un reacted oils in the cleaning soap, enhancing its conditioning impact.

3. Add Humectant:

- Include ingredients like glycerin, honey, or aloe vera juice on your soap recipe to draw moisture to the pores and skin and improve hydration.

BALANCING LATHERING:

1. Incorporate Lathering Oils:

- Include oils and fat that contribute to a rich and stable lather. Examples consist of coconut oil, palm oil, and babassu oil.

- Use oils high in lauric acid for a bubbly lather and oils high in stearic acid for a creamy lather.

2. Consider Soap Formulation:

- Adjust the ratio of difficult oils (which make contributions to lather) and gentle oils (which make contributions to conditioning) primarily based to your desired lathering effect.

3. Additives for Lather:

- Include components like sodium lactate or sugar on your recipe to decorate lather balance and richness.

TESTING AND ADJUSTING:

1. Small Batch Testing:

- Make a small batch of your soap recipe to test its cleaning, moisturizing, and lathering houses.

- Evaluate the cleaning soap's performance throughout use, along with its cleansing energy, moisturizing sense, and lather satisfactory.

2. Gather Feedback:

- Gather remarks from testers or users to recognize how the soap performs on special pores and skin types and in numerous situations.

- Use feedback to make adjustments on your recipe, which includes tweaking oil chances, superfat levels, or components.

3. Iterate and Refine:

- Continuously iterate and refine your cleaning soap recipes primarily based on testing effects and person feedback to attain the desired balance of homes.

USING A SOAP CALCULATOR

Using a cleaning soap calculator is a important step in formulating soap recipes accurately and competently. Soap calculators assist determine the proper amounts of oils, lye, water, and components needed for a balanced and lye safe cleaning soap recipe.

Step 1: Choose a Soap Calculator

1. Online Calculators:

- There are numerous free and reliable soap calculators to be had online, inclusive of Soap Calc, Bramble Berry's

Lye Calculator, and Majestic Mountain Sage's Lye Calculator.

- Choose a calculator that offers distinctive statistics, which includes fatty acid profiles, endorsed usage charges for components, and lye concentration alternatives.

2. Downloadable Software:

- Some soap makers decide upon downloadable cleaning soap calculators for offline use. Examples consist of Soap Maker and Soap Calc for Windows.

Step 2: Input Recipe Details

1. Select Measurement Units:

- Choose among oz (ounces), grams (g), pounds (lb), or other favored gadgets for measuring substances.

2. Enter Oil/Fat Percentages:

- Input the percentages of each oil or fat you want to consist of on your soap recipe. Ensure the whole adds up to one hundred%.

3. Set Super fat Percentage:

● Determine the super fat percentage, which is the quantity of unreacted oils left in the cleaning soap for delivered moisturizing. Common super fat probabilities range from five% to eight%.

4. Choose Lye Concentration:

● Select the lye concentration based totally to your preferred cleaning soap houses. Higher lye concentration effects in a extra cleaning cleaning soap, while lower attention yields a milder cleaning soap.

● Typical lye awareness alternatives include 28% for a moderate cleaning soap, 3033% for a balanced soap, and 38% for a cleaning cleaning soap.

5. Enter Additives (Optional):

- If including components such as important oils, fragrances, colorants, or botanical, input their possibilities or amounts into the calculator.

- Follow encouraged usage quotes for additives to make certain protection and effectiveness.

Step 3: Calculate and Review Results

1. Click Calculate:

- Once you've entered all recipe information, click the calculate or generate button at the cleaning soap calculator.

2. Review Recipe Details:

- Review the calculated recipe info provided by way of the calculator, including:

Amounts of oils, lye, and water wanted.

PRACTICE EXAMPLES.

Sure, permit's go through multiple practice examples the usage of a cleaning soap calculator. We'll create exceptional soap recipes with various residences.

Example 1: Moisturizing and Conditioning Soap

- Objective: Creatc a gentle and moisturizing cleaning soap appropriate for dry and sensitive skin.

- Ingredients:

- Olive Oil: 40%

- Coconut Oil: 25%

- Shea Butter: 20%

- Castor Oil: 10%

- Sweet Almond Oil: 5%

- Super fat: 5%

- Fragrance (nonobligatory): 1 ounces consistent with pound of oils

INSTRUCTIONS:

1. Go to a cleaning soap calculator like Soap Calc.

2. Choose the devices of dimension (oz, grams, kilos).

3. Input the chances of every oil: Olive Oil (forty%), Coconut Oil (25%), Shea Butter (20%), Castor Oil (10%), Sweet Almond Oil (five%).

Four. Set the super fat percent to 5%.

5. Enter any extra additives or perfume if preferred.

6. Click "Calculate" to generate the recipe.

RESULTS:

- Total oil weight: one thousand grams
- Lye (Sodium Hydroxide) required: 139 grams
- Water required: 318 grams
- Super fat: 5%
- Estimated residences: Gentle cleansing, excessive conditioning, creamy lather

Adjust the perfume amount based totally in your preference and the producer's guidelines.

Example 2: Cleansing and Refreshing Soap

● Objective: Create a soap with strong cleansing houses and a refreshing heady scent.

● Ingredients:

● Coconut Oil: 50%

● Palm Oil: 30%

● Olive Oil: 10%

● Castor Oil: five%

● Peppermint Essential Oil: 2 ouncesin line with pound of oils

● Super fat: five%

Instructions:

1. Use the same cleaning soap calculator and units of measurement.

2. Input the percentages of each oil: Coconut Oil (50%), Palm Oil (30%), Olive Oil (10%), Castor Oil (five%)

3. Set the super fat percentage to five%.

4. Add Peppermint Essential Oil at 2 ounce sin line with pound of oils.

Five. Click "Calculate" to generate the recipe.

Results:

 Total oil weight: 1000 grams

 Lye (Sodium Hydroxide) required: 127 grams

 Water required: 292 grams

 Super fat: five%

 Estimated homes: Strong cleaning, fresh fragrance, appropriate lather

Adjust the amount of vital oil primarily based in your preference for fragrance power.

CHAPTER 6: COLORING AND SCENTING YOUR SOAP

NATURAL COLORANTS

HERBS, CLAY, AND OTHER HERBAL ADDITIVES.

Certainly! Herbs, clay, and other natural additives can beautify the residences and visual enchantment of home made soap.

HERBS:

1. Selection:

- Choose dried herbs based on their homes and desired outcomes. For example, lavender for rest, calendula for soothing homes, or peppermint for a refreshing scent.

- Ensure herbs are thoroughly dried to save you mold inside the cleaning soap.

2. Preparation:

- Crush or grind dried herbs into smaller pieces to facilitate even distribution within the soap.

- Infuse herbs in a provider oil (like olive oil) in advance for a more reported herbal fragrance and benefits.

3. Incorporation:

- Add herbs to the cleaning soap combination at hint (for bloodless process) or while the soap base has cooled slightly (for soften and pour).

- Stir herbs lightly into the cleaning soap combination to distribute calmly.

4. Amount:

- Use around 12 tablespoons of dried herbs in line with pound of cleaning soap base. Adjust based totally at the herb's efficiency and desired concentration in the cleaning soap.

Clay:

1. Selection:

- Choose cosmetic grade clay together with kaolin clay, French green clay, bentonite clay, or rhassoul clay.

- Each clay has extraordinary homes (e.G., kaolin for gentle cleaning, bentonite for detoxing), so pick out based for your goals.

2. Preparation:

- Mix clay with a small quantity of water or liquid oil (from your soap recipe) to create a clean paste earlier than including it to the soap aggregate.

- Avoid including dry clay at once to the cleaning soap as it could motive clumping.

3. Incorporation:

- Add clay paste to the cleaning soap mixture at hint (for bloodless technique) or when the soap base has cooled slightly (for soften and pour).

Stir properly to make certain the clay is evenly distributed.

4. Amount:

- Use 12 tablespoons of clay according to pound of cleaning soap base. Adjust based totally on the desired shade and properties of the soap.

OTHER NATURAL ADDITIVES:

1. Essential Oils:

- Choose highquality critical oils for heady scent and capability healing advantages.

- Add critical oils at trace for cold system cleaning soap or while the cleaning soap base has cooled for melt and pour.

2. Exfoliants:

Include natural exfoliants like floor oats, coffee grounds, poppy seeds, or finely ground nuts for gentle exfoliation.

ESSENTIAL OILS AND FRAGRANCES

Essential oils and fragrances are key components in soap making, including fragrance, therapeutic benefits, and attraction for your creations.

ESSENTIAL OILS:

1. Selection:

- Choose exquisite, natural important oils from professional providers. Consider the fragrance profile and ability healing residences of every oil.
- Popular crucial oils for soap making encompass lavender, tea tree, eucalyptus, peppermint, citrus oils (orange, lemon), and floral oils (rose, jasmine).

2. Usage Rates:

- Essential oils are effective, so use them sparingly. Generally, the endorsed utilization price is zero.Five3% of the total soap batch weight.

- Calculate the quantity of critical oil wanted primarily based on the favored heady scent energy and the full weight of oils to your cleaning soap recipe.

3. Addition Time:

- Add vital oils to the cleaning soap mixture at trace (for cold process) or whilst the cleaning soap base has cooled barely (for soften and pour).

- Stir gently but thoroughly to ensure even distribution of the important oils at some stage in the cleaning soap.

4. Therapeutic Benefits:

- Each important oil has unique therapeutic blessings. For instance, lavender promotes relaxation, tea tree has antimicrobial properties, and peppermint offers a cooling sensation.

- Consider the intended use of the cleaning soap (e.G., frame soap, facial soap) and choose critical oils that align with those functions.

FRAGRANCE OILS:

1. Selection:

- Fragrance oils are synthetic or natural blends designed to feature heady scent to cleaning soap. Choose outstanding fragrance oils which might be pores and skin secure and in particular formulated for soap making.

- Fragrance oils provide a huge range of scents, from fruity and floral to woodsy and highly spiced.

2. Usage Rates:

- Follow the producer's pointers for perfume oil utilization fees, typically round 1five% of the entire soap batch weight.

- Calculate the quantity of fragrance oil wished primarily based on the advocated usage fee and your preferred fragrance strength.

3. Stability:

- Fragrance oils regularly have better fragrance retention than critical oils in cleaning soap. They can provide long lasting perfume even after curing.

- Test fragrances in small batches to ensure they carry out well in soap and keep their scent over the years.

4. Blending:

- Create custom fragrance blends via combining more than one important oils or fragrance oils. Experiment with one of a kind mixtures to achieve precise scents.

- Keep music of your fragrance blends and their ratios for destiny reference and consistency.

SAFETY CONSIDERATIONS:

1. Skin Sensitivity:

- Some vital oils and perfume oils may additionally cause skin irritation or sensitization in ccrtain people. Always carry out a patch take a look at earlier than using a new oil.

- Use caution with oils regarded to be photo toxic (e.G., citrus oils) and follow encouraged utilization recommendations.

2. Allergies:

- Be mindful of capacity allergic reactions to particular essential oils or perfume additives. Label your cleaning soap elements really for patron consciousness.

3. Storage:

- Store crucial oils and perfume oils in dark ish, cool locations far from daylight and heat to hold their scent and excellent.

- Keep bottles tightly closed to prevent evaporation and oxidation.

BENEFITS OF THE USE OF ESSENTIAL OILS.

Using crucial oils in cleaning soap making gives various benefits, which include aromatic attraction, capability therapeutic homes, and natural upgrades to the soap's features.

AROMATIC APPEAL:

1. Natural Scents:

- Essential oils offer natural and natural scents derived from botanical resources. They offer a wide range of fragrances, from floral and fruity to woody and natural, improving the sensory enjoy of the use of the cleaning soap.

2. Customization:

- Create custom heady scent blends by means of combining exclusive essential oils. This lets in you to tailor the aroma of your cleaning soap to in shape various preferences and activities.

3. Long Lasting Fragrance:

- Some critical oils have awesome scent retention homes, providing long lasting fragrance in cleaning soap even after curing. They can contribute to a nice and lasting aroma at some point of use.

THERAPEUTIC PROPERTIES:

1. Aromatherapy Benefits:

- Certain essential oils have therapeutic homes that could definitely impact temper and emotions. For instance, lavender promotes relaxation, whilst peppermint gives a refreshing and invigorating heady scent.

2. Skin Benefits:

- Some important oils have skin nourishing residences, together with tea tree oil's antimicrobial consequences or chamomile oil's soothing houses. Incorporating those oils into soap can gain the pores and skin at some point of cleansing.

3. Potential Healing Effects:

- Essential oils like eucalyptus or tea tree oil are acknowledged for his or her antibacterial and anti fungal homes, which can help deal with pores and skin problems like acne or minor pores and skin irritations.

Natural Enhancements to Soap:

1. Antioxidant Properties:

- Certain critical oils, consisting of rosemary or citrus oils, include antioxidants that can assist defend the skin from environmental damage and sell skin health.

2. Moisturizing Effects:

- Some important oils, like geranium or jojoba oil, have moisturizing and hydrating houses. When used in cleaning soap, they are able to contribute to a softer and more nourished pores and skin experience.

3. Anti inflammatory Benefits:

- Essential oils which include chamomile or lavender have anti inflammatory properties which can help soothe indignant or infected skin, making them beneficial for sensitive pores and skin sorts.

4. Natural Preservation:

- Certain important oils, like tea tree oil or rosemary oil, have herbal preservative residences that could assist increase the shelf existence of cleaning soap by using inhibiting microbial growth.

Environmentally Friendly:

1. Biodegradable:

- Essential oils are derived from herbal plant assets and are biodegradable, making them environmentally friendly as compared to artificial fragrances.

BLENDING ESSENTIAL OILS.

Blending vital oils is an clever manner that permits you to create custom scents tailored for your alternatives or particular therapeutic dreams.

1. Understand Essential Oil Notes:

Top Notes: These are the first scents you understand and tend to be mild, fresh, and uplifting. Examples encompass citrus oils (e.G., lemon, orange), peppermint, and eucalyptus.

- Middle Notes (Heart Notes): These scents emerge after the pinnacle notes and are frequently floral, natural, or fruity. Examples include lavender, geranium, rosemary, and chamomile.

- Base Notes: These scents are deep, wealthy, and long lasting, supplying a solid foundation to the blend. Examples encompass patchouli, sandalwood, cedar wood, and vanilla.

2. Consider Scent Profiles:

- Harmonious Blends: Choose oils that supplement each different to create a balanced and harmonious heady scent. For instance, pair citrus oils with floral or herbal oils for a clean mixture.

- Contrasting Blends: Experiment with contrasting scents to create particular and dynamic blends. Combine floral and spicy oils or citrus and woody oils for complexity.

3. Start with Small Batches:

Begin with the aid of blending small quantities of essential oils, especially in case you're experimenting with new combos. This lets in you to alter the ratios without difficulty and avoid losing oils.

4. Keep Track of Ratios:

Use a dropper or pipette to measure the drops of each critical oil correctly. Keep tune of the ratios utilized in a hit blends for future reference.

5. Test Blends:

- Perform a fragrance check by putting a drop of the blend on a scent strip or for your wrist. Allow the combination to evolve and notice how the special notes engage over the years.

- Evaluate the combo's average heady scent, balance, and the way it makes you sense. Consider how the combo can be used (e.G., in soap, diffuser, rubdown oil) while assessing its effectiveness.

6. Adjust and Refine:

- If a mix is simply too overpowering or lacks complexity, adjust the ratios with the aid of including more of the bottom, center, or top notes accordingly.

- Take notes during the mixing method to report a success blends and any adjustments made. This facilitates in refining your blending talents through the years.

RECOMMENDED AMOUNTS AND SAFETY RECOMMENDATIONS.

When mixing essential oils to be used in soap making or different applications, it is vital to follow endorsed amounts and protection guidelines to ensure effectiveness and limit the hazard of negative reactions.

RECOMMENDED AMOUNTS:

1. Usage Rates:

- For cleaning soap making, the typical utilization charge of important oils is round zero.Five% to three% of the overall weight of oils to your soap recipe.

- Example: If your soap batch weighs 1000 grams (overall oils), the amount of vital oil ought to be between 5 to 30 grams (zero.5% to a few%).

2. Scent Strength:

- Start with smaller amounts of important oils and alter based totally at the preferred fragrance power. Some oils are effective, and a bit is going a long manner.

- Keep in mind that sure vital oils have stronger scents and can require decrease quantities to reap the desired fragrance.

SAFETY GUIDELINES:

1. Skin Sensitivity:

- Perform a patch take a look at earlier than the usage of a new critical oil, specially if you have sensitive pores and skin or allergic reactions.

- Dilute vital oils nicely in carrier oils (e.G., olive oil, candy almond oil) whilst the usage of them without delay at the pores and skin or in soap to lessen the hazard of infection.

2. Photo toxicity:

- Some citrus essential oils (e.G., lemon, lime, bergamot) are photo toxic, that means they could motive pores and skin sensitivity and reactions when uncovered to daylight.

- Use photo toxic oils in low concentrations and avoid direct solar exposure after application.

3. Pregnancy and Children:

- Consult with a healthcare expert earlier than the usage of critical oils, especially in the course of pregnancy, breastfeeding, or with younger kids.

- Some essential oils are not recommended for use for the duration of pregnancy or might also require dilution for safe use.

4. Storage and Handling:

- Store critical oils in dark ish, glass bottles away from sunlight and warmth to hold their efficiency and high quality.

- Keep essential oils out of attain of kids and pets, as they're concentrated and may be dangerous if ingested.

5. Labeling:

- Clearly label your vital oil blends and merchandise with the names and probabilities of important oils used.

CHAPTER 7: ADVANCED TECHNIQUES AND TIPS

SWIRLING AND LAYERING

Techniques for creating beautiful designs. Creating stunning designs in cleaning soap making includes various techniques that upload visual enchantment and creativity to your finished merchandise.

1. Swirling Techniques:

- Drop Swirl: Pour different coloured soap batter in a circular pattern, creating a drop impact when mixed.

- In The Pot Swirl: Swirl exclusive coloured batters inside the soap pot earlier than pouring into molds, creating complex patterns.

- Linear Swirl: Pour alternating colour of cleaning soap batter in a straight line, then use a tool to create swirls.

2. Layering Techniques:

- Vertical Layering: Pour layers of in a different way colored or scented soap batter vertically inside the mold for a layered effect.
- Horizontal Layering: Pour layers of soap batter horizontally, growing distinct layers seen at the soap's cut surface.

3. Embeds and Inclusions:

- Embed small cleaning soap shapes (e.G., hearts, flowers) within a larger soap batch for delivered interest and dimension.
- Include herbal exfoliants (e.G., oats, poppy seeds) or decorative elements (e.G., dried plants, herbs) in cleaning soap layers for texture and visual appeal.

4. Texture Techniques:

- Texture Tops: Use a spatula, spoon, or comb to create textured styles on the pinnacle floor of the cleaning soap.

- Salt or Sugar Crystals: Sprinkle coarse salt or sugar crystals on the soap surface for a sparkling impact.

- Drag Swirls: Drag a skewer or toothpick via the cleaning soap batter to create swirls or patterns.

5. Color Techniques:

- Natural Colorants: Use natural colorants like clay, botanical powders, or natural infusions to create earthy tones and diffused sun shades.

- Mica Powders: Add shimmer and sparkle to soap designs using mica powders in diverse colour.

- Layered Colors: Pour layers of in a different way coloured cleaning soap batter to create vibrant and colourful designs.

6. Advanced Techniques:

- CPOP (Cold Process Oven Process): Heat cleaning soap inside the oven after molding to accelerate saponification and create vibrant shades and swirls.

- Fluid Pouring: Pour soap batter from exceptional heights or angles to create particular styles and designs.

TIPS FOR DESIGN SUCCESS:

1. Plan Ahead: Sketch out your layout ideas and plan the colors, layers, and strategies you'll use earlier than beginning.

2. Use Quality Ingredients: Use great oils, colorants, and fragrances to make sure vibrant shades and long lasting scents.

3. Work at Optimal Temperatures: Soap batter should be at a medium trace consistency for most designs, taking into account manipulation with out becoming too thick.

4. Practice Patience: Allow layers to set earlier than including the next layer or layout detail to save you mixing and smudging.

5. Experiment and Have Fun: Don't be afraid to attempt new techniques and mixtures. Soap making is an art, and creativity often ends in lovely effects!

EMBEDDING AND TEXTURING

Embedding and texturing are creative strategies which could upload intensity, hobby, and uniqueness on your handmade soaps.

Embedding:

1. Select Embeds:

- Choose small cleaning soap shapes or items to embed inside your cleaning soap bars. These can include hearts, stars, plants, seashells, or even small soap cubes.

2. Prepare Embeds:

- Create the embeds using a separate cleaning soap batch or leftover cleaning soap scraps. Pour the cleaning soap into small molds or reduce it into desired shapes once it has cooled and hardened.

3. Embedding Process:

- Pour a thin layer of plain cleaning soap batter into the cleaning soap mold, protecting the lowest.

- Place the embeds onto the poured layer of cleaning soap. Arrange them lightly or in a desired sample.

- Pour the remaining cleaning soap batter over the embeds, ensuring they're absolutely blanketed and secured inside the cleaning soap.

4. Tips for Embedding:

- Ensure the embeds are absolutely cured and organization earlier than embedding them in the soap to prevent them from melting or distorting.

- Use a spatula or skewer to softly press down on the embeds to ensure they're

fully embedded and surrounded via
cleaning soap.

TEXTURING:

1. Texture Tools:

● Use a variety of tools to create textured styles on the floor of the soap. These can consist of spatulas, forks, combs, wood skewers, or even natural substances like leaves or shells.

2. Texture Techniques:

● Drag Swirls: Drag a skewer or comb via the cleaning soap batter in a swirling motion to create swirls or patterns.

● Spatter Effect: Splatter small droplets of colored cleaning soap batter onto the soap surface the usage of a broom or toothbrush for a speckled effect.

● Textured Tops: Use a spatula or textured device to create peaks, waves, or ridges on the top floor of the cleaning soap.

- Stamping: Press textured stamps or gadgets onto the cleaning soap surface earlier than it units to create imprints and patterns.

3. Layering with Texture:

- Incorporate textured layers inside the cleaning soap by means of pouring specific colored or textured cleaning soap batters in layers. Drag a device through the layers to create precise designs.

4. Tips for Texturing:

- Work fast but cautiously while texturing to avoid over blending or blending the cleaning soap layers.

- Experiment with one of a kind tools and techniques to create a variety of textures and designs.

SAFETY CONSIDERATIONS:

Ensure that any gear or items used for embedding or texturing are clean and clean up to maintain cleaning soap hygiene.

ADDING BOTANICAL AND TEXTURES.

Adding botanical and textures to home made soap can raise its visual attraction and provide particular sensory experiences.

BOTANICAL:

1. Selection of Botanical:

Choose dried botanical which are suitable to be used in soap, which includes dried flowers (e.G., lavender buds, calendula petals), herbs (e.G., rosemary, chamomile), or seeds (e.G., poppy seeds, chia seeds).

● Ensure botanical are very well dried to save you mould formation inside the soap.

2. Preparation:

- Crush or grind large botanical into smaller pieces to facilitate even distribution inside the cleaning soap.

- Infuse botanical in a service oil (e.G., olive oil) in advance to extract their herbal colour and houses for a greater suggested effect.

3. Incorporation:

- Add botanical to the soap combination at trace (for bloodless process) or whilst the cleaning soap base has cooled barely (for melt and pour).

- Gently stir botanical into the soap aggregate to distribute flippantly. Avoid over mixing to prevent color bleeding or choppy distribution.

4. Placement:

- Sprinkle botanical on pinnacle of the soap combination inside the mold for a ornamental touch. Press them lightly into

the floor to ensure they adhere to the
cleaning soap.

5. Amount:

- Use botanical sparsely to keep away
from an overly textured or abrasive
cleaning soap. Aim for a balanced
appearance with seen botanical however
no longer overwhelming.

TEXTURES:

1. Tools for Texturing:

- Utilize numerous equipment and
techniques to create textures at the soap's
floor. Examples encompass spatulas,
forks, combs, wood skewers, textured
stamps, or natural substances like leaves
or shells.

2. Texturing Techniques:

- Drag Swirls: Drag a skewer or comb
thru the cleaning soap batter in swirling
motions to create swirls or styles.

- Spatter Effect: Splatter small droplets of colored soap batter onto the soap floor using a brush or toothbrush for a speckled impact.

- Texture Tops: Use a spatula or textured device to create peaks, waves, or ridges at the top floor of the soap.

- Stamping: Press textured stamps or gadgets onto the cleaning soap surface before it sets to create imprints and styles.

3. Layering with Texture:

- Incorporate textured layers within the soap through pouring exclusive coloured or textured soap batters in layers. Drag a device through the layers to create particular designs.

4. Natural Textures:

- Consider the usage of herbal substances like oatmeal, espresso grounds, pumice powder, or clays (e.G.,

kaolin, French green clay) to feature
texture and exfoliation houses to the
soap.

SAFETY CONSIDERATIONS:

- Ensure that any botanical or herbal
  textures used are clean, dry, and loose
  from contaminants to maintain cleaning
  soap hygienc.

- Test botanical and textures in small
  batches to study how they interact with
  the soap base and how they have an
  effect on the very last look and feel of
  the soap.

CHAPTER 8: CURING, STORING, AND PACKAGING

CURING YOUR SOAP

WHY CURING IS IMPORTANT.

Curing is an important step in the cleaning soap making method that involves permitting the freshly made cleaning soap to undergo a length of rest and drying before it is ready for use.

1. Hardening and Stabilization:

- Curing permits the soap to harden and stabilize over the years. During the curing technique, excess water evaporates from the soap, resulting in a less attachable and longer lasting bar.

2. Improved Lather and Mildness:

- Cured soap produces a richer and creamier lather in comparison to freshly made soap. This superior lather enjoy contributes to a extra enjoyable cleaning enjoy.

- The curing procedure also allows the soap to grow to be milder and gentler at the pores and skin. It gives the soap time to finish the saponification reaction, lowering the presence of caustic lye within the very last product.

3. Reduction of Water Content:

- As the cleaning soap remedies, its water content material decreases. This discount in water content leads to a denser and harder bar, making it less prone to melting and ensuring it lasts longer in use.

4. Enhanced Fragrance:

- Cured soap frequently develops a more pronounced and well rounded fragrance compared to freshly made cleaning soap. The curing length lets in the scent to mature and stabilize within the soap, resulting in a longer lasting aroma.

5. Reduction of pH:

- The curing technique contributes to a reduction inside the soap's pH stage, making it milder and extra suitable for sensitive pores and skin.

- Freshly made soap may have a higher pH because of the presence of unreacted lye, which can be harsh at the skin. Curing helps stability and neutralize the pH over time.

6. Increased Hardness and Longevity:

- Cured soap is harder and less probably to dissolve speedy in water. This multiplied hardness improves the soap's durability and sturdiness, making it extra low in cost for use.

PROPER CURING SITUATIONS.

Proper curing situations are vital for reaching the excellent effects while curing handmade soap.

1. Air Circulation:

- Place the soap bars on a drying rack or tray with a space between each bar to allow for most desirable air circulation. Avoid stacking the bars at once on pinnacle of each different, as this could restrict airflow and slow down the curing manner.

2. Temperature and Humidity:

- Curing ought to take vicinity in a groovy, dry environment with steady room temperature. Avoid exposing the soap to excessive temperatures, direct daylight, or excessive humidity, as those factors can affect the soap's texture, colour, and perfume.

3. Ventilation:

- Ensure the curing region is nicely ventilated to save you moisture buildup across the soap bars. Good ventilation helps facilitate the evaporation of excess water from the cleaning soap, leading to less assailable and longer lasting bars.

4. Drying Time:

- The advocated curing time for home made cleaning soap is usually four to 6 weeks, despite the fact that positive recipes may also gain from longer curing periods. Allow enough time for the cleaning soap to dry and harden absolutely before use.

5. Rotation:

Periodically rotate the soap bars at some stage in the curing method to make sure even drying and prevent flat spots or indentations on the lowest of the bars. This also allows sell uniform texture and consistency across all bars.

6. Protection from Contaminants:

- Keep the curing region smooth and unfastened from dust, debris, or contaminants that may come into touch with the cleaning soap bars. Cover the soap bars with a breathable fabric (e.G., paper or cloth) to protect them even as allowing airflow.

7. Monitoring:

- Regularly inspect the soap bars at some stage in the curing length for any signs and symptoms of moisture or sweating. If you observe any moisture buildup, retain curing the bars till they are completely dry and firm to the touch.

STORING YOUR SOAP

Proper storage is prime to retaining the great, freshness, and longevity of your handcrafted soap.

1. Cool, Dry Location:

- Store your soap in a fab, dry place far from direct daylight, warmness sources, and humidity. Excessive warmth and moisture can cause the soap to soften, melt, or develop sweat beads (glycerin dew).

2. Air Circulation:

- Provide good enough air stream around the soap bars to save you moisture buildup. Avoid tightly wrapping the cleaning soap in airtight packing containers or plastic wrap, as this will entice moisture and have an effect on the cleaning soap's texture.

3. Elevated Surface:

- Place the soap bars on a raised or slatted floor, inclusive of a drying rack or soap dish, to permit air to circulate around the bottom of the bars. This helps save you the soap from turning into soggy or sticking to surfaces.

4. Avoid Damp Areas:

- Keep cleaning soap far from areas at risk of moisture, which include toilets with frequent showers or steam. Moisture publicity can cause the cleaning soap to soften and lose its hardness through the years.

5. Use Breathable Packaging:

- If storing soap in bins or packaging, select breathable materials consisting of paper luggage, cardboard bins, or fabric pouches. These materials allow air to glide around the soap at the same time as defensive it from dust and particles.

- Ideal garage conditions to maintain best. To hold the best, freshness, and durability of your handcrafted cleaning soap, it is vital to shop it underneath best conditions. Here are the proper storage situations to hold the exceptional of your cleaning soap:

1. Temperature:

- Ideal Temperature Range: Store cleaning soap in a place where temperatures are constant and variety among 50°F to 70°F (10°C to 21°C).

- Avoid Extreme Temperatures: Keep soap away from direct daylight, warmness sources, and cold drafts, as extreme temperatures can affect the texture, scent, and coloration of the cleaning soap.

2. Humidity:

- Low Humidity: Store soap in a low humidity surroundings to save you excess moisture absorption, which could lead to softening, sweating, or mildew boom.

- Avoid Damp Areas: Keep soap away from lavatories or areas with high humidity degrees, such as close to sinks or showers.

3. Air Circulation:

- Adequate Airflow: Provide enough air stream around the cleaning soap bars to permit them to respire and save you moisture buildup.

- Elevated Storage: Use slatted cleaning soap dishes, drying racks, or trays to raise soap bars and sell airflow under.

4. Light:

- Avoid Direct Sunlight: Store cleaning soap far from direct sunlight or excessive synthetic mild, as UV rays can fade colour and degrade fragrances over time.

- Use Opaque Packaging: If the usage of boxes, opt for opaque or tinted substances to defend soap from light publicity.

5. Packaging:

- Breathable Materials: Store soap in breathable packaging, such as paper bags, cardboard boxes, or cloth pouches, to allow air stream even as defensive it from dust and particles.

- Avoid Airtight Containers: Do no longer save soap in airtight containers or plastic wrap, as this may entice moisture and have an effect on the cleaning soap's texture and heady scent.

6. Labeling and Rotation:

- Labeling: Label each batch of cleaning soap with the date of manufacturing and curing time to tune freshness and usage order.

- Rotation: Use older batches of soap first to hold freshness and ensure consistent satisfactory across batches.

7. Fragrance Protection:

● Separate Strong Scents: Store soap away from sturdy smelling objects or chemical substances to prevent perfume transfer and hold the soap's authentic scent.

8. Storage Location:

● Cool, Dry Area: Choose a fab, dry place in your own home for cleaning soap garage, consisting of a linen closet, pantry, or bedroom drawer.

● Avoid Moisture Sources: Keep soap away from sinks, water warmers, or areas susceptible to water leaks to prevent unintentional moisture publicity.

ECO FRIENDLY PACKAGING OPTIONS.

When it involves packaging handmade cleaning soap in an eco friendly way, there are several options you may take into account.

1. Recycled Paper or Cardboard:

- Kraft Paper Wrappers: Wrap individual cleaning soap bars in unbleached kraft paper or recycled paper wrappers. These wrappers are biodegradable and can be composted.

- Cardboard Boxes: Use cardboard containers made from recycled substances to bundle multiple cleaning soap bars. Opt for containers with minimum or no plastic coatings.

2. Biodegradable or Compo-stable Materials:

- Biodegradable Plastic Wraps: If you choose to use wraps, pick out biodegradable or compo stable plastic wraps made from plant based totally substances like PLA (poly lactic acid) or cellulose.

- Cornstarch Based Bags: Package soap bars in biodegradable baggage crafted from cornstarch or different natural substances. These luggage spoil down easily in composting situations.

3. Glass or Metal Containers:

Glass Jars: Package liquid or whipped soap in reusable glass jars with metal lids. Glass is recyclable, and reusable jars reduce unmarried use packaging waste.

Metal Tins: Use metallic tins or containers made from aluminum or tinplate for stable bar soaps. These tins are long lasting and recyclable.

4. Cloth or Fabric Wraps:

Fabric Bags: Wrap soap bars in material baggage or pouches made from cotton, linen, or other herbal fibers. Fabric wraps may be reused or repurposed through customers.

Beeswax Wraps: Consider using beeswax wraps as an opportunity to plastic wraps for packaging. These wraps are reusable and biodegradable.

5. Paperboard Packaging:

- Paperboard Boxes: Choose paperboard packing containers made from recycled materials for packaging gift units or special cleaning soap collections. Look for packing containers with soy based inks and minimum plastic inserts.

- Seed Paper Inserts: Include seed paper inserts inner packaging that customers can plant to grow wildflowers or herbs. Seed paper is biodegradable and adds a sustainable touch.

LABELING NECESSITIES AND RECOMMENDATIONS.

Labeling requirements for handmade cleaning soap range relying for your location and the regulations set by using relevant authorities. It's essential to comply with labeling requirements to make sure transparency, protection, and legal compliance.

1. Product Name:

Include the call of your soap product
prominently on the label. This might be a
innovative or descriptive call that displays
the cleaning soap's substances, perfume, or
blessings.

2. Ingredients List:

Provide an in depth listing of all substances
used within the cleaning soap, which include
botanical, vital oils, colorants, and
components. List substances in descending
order of predominance by using weight.

Use INCI (International Nomenclature of
Cosmetic Ingredients) names for elements to
make certain readability and consistency.

3. Net Weight or Volume:

Clearly nation the net weight (for solid
soaps) or extent (for liquid soaps) of the
product on the label. This enables clients
recognize the quantity they're shopping.

4. Batch Code or Number:

 Assign a batch code or variety to each production batch of soap. This permits for traceability in case of nice manipulate or remember problems.

 5. Manufacturer Information:

Include your business name, cope with, and call facts on the label. This identifies the manufacturer or supplier of the cleaning soap and offers contact details for clients.